DISEASE BELIEFS IN MEXICAN-AMERICAN COMMUNITIES

LINDA C. ROSE

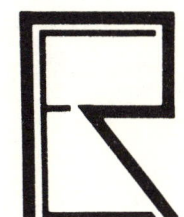

San Francisco, California
1978

Published By

R & E RESEARCH ASSOCIATES, INC.
4843 Mission Street
San Francisco, California 94112

Publishers

Robert D. Reed and Adam S. Eterovich

Library of Congress Card Catalog Number

77-90359

I.S.B.N.

0-88247-519-3

ACKNOWLEDGEMENTS

I want to take this opportunity to thank professors Robert Ravicz, Lynn Mason, and Keith Morton for their many helpful comments and assistance on this project.

I also wish to thank my husband, Robert M. Rose and D. and S. Poster for their patience and unstinting help.

TABLE OF CONTENTS

LIST OF TABLES

VII

CHAPTER I

INTRODUCTION

Background

A survey of the literature on Mexican-American disease
and health beliefs between 1945 and 1975 emphasizes the
changes in approaches used by anthropologists, in particular
and by social scientists, in general. The earlier work done
between 1945 and 1965 examines disease and health beliefs
through descriptive studies of small, autonomous units. These
studies are based on fieldwork with participant observation.
Hypotheses are suggested but not tested in a statistical or
quantitative way.

During the middle and late 1960's, anthropology and
other disciplines within the social sciences began to test
and quantify Mexican-American behaviors and attitudes towards
health care. For the most part, this was carried out in
urban areas while the earlier, ethnographic studies were done
in more rural sectors.

In 1957, Rubel (1960:814) studied changing concepts of
disease and health among Mexican-Americans in a town in
Hidalgo County, Texas. The population of 15,000 included
9,000 Mexican-American residents. In this study, Rubel
derived the following hypothesis: "the greater the number

of Mexican-Americans who adopt new behavior and values; the more value will the traditionally-oriented invest in the aggregate of caida de mollera (fallen fontanel), empacho (surfeit), mal de ojo (evil eye), and susto (fright, soul loss)." These are four folk disease categories which Rubel hypothesized present a hard core of resistance to modern medical practices because they support certain "core values" and ways of behavior in a Mexican-American Community. Rubel's underlying assumption appears to be that the more Mexican-Americans become acculturated, the more the traditionally-oriented will cling to folk disease beliefs.

In a later work, Rubel (1966:195) again hypothesized that some Mexican-Americans associated folk disease beliefs with resistance to acculturation or what Farge (1975:31) termed, "resistance to anglicization". According to Rubel (1966:195), "The unusual acclaim awarded each victory of a traditional means of healing can be understood as an effort to validate the worth of the traditional culture in face of constant and severe criticism by Anglos especially in the area of health-related beliefs and behavior."

Along with the above hypothesis that retention of folk disease concepts by traditionally-oriented Mexican-Americans is related to resistance to anglicization, Rubel (1966:xxii) also contended that the social and belief systems of Mexican-Americans "impede full utilization of available professional health services."

Goals

The primary aim of this study is to examine Rubel's two related hypotheses which he derived from non-urban populations in south Texas. In order to do this, the hypotheses are broken down into three questions which are addressed within the confines of this paper.

1. Do Mexican-American folk disease concepts support traditional core values of the social system.

2. Do traditionally-oriented Mexican-Americans retain beliefs in the four folk diseases (susto, caida de mollera, empacho, and mal de ojo) and is this associated with resistance to anglicization? A fifth diagnostic category, mal puesto (diseases caused by witchcraft) is added because of the importance not only in Rubel's studies (1962, 1966) but in much of the literature.

3. Is retention of folk disease beliefs associated with underutilization of professional (scientific or Anglo) health services?

The terms used in these questions are defined for use in this paper as follows:

1. core values - These values are shared by the whole group and are necessary for the smooth functioning of social relations. Mexican-American core values include: the importance of the three generation family of socialization, the importance of the older over the younger, and men over women (Rubel 1960:809-811). Another core value is what

3

Madsen (1964:44) terms, "the family as a sanctuary in a hostile world".

2. <u>underutilization</u> - Proportionately less use of professional health care services than either Anglo or other ethnic or minority groups.

3. <u>Mexican-American</u> - The population under study includes those individuals of Mexican ancestry born in the United States of residents of the United States who were born in Mexico. The population included in the literature used for this study, reside in the Southwestern part of the United States. There are two exceptions: Nebraska (Welch, Comer and Steinman, 1973) and Detroit (Humphrey:1945). In this study, the Southwest includes the states of Arizona, California, Colorado, New Mexico, and Texas.

Besides answering the three questions, a concomitant goal of this study is to correlate data about Mexican-American disease concepts which up to very recent times have rarely been compared.

Creson, McKinley and Evans (1969:266) suggest that the whole area of folk disease beliefs has not been comprehensively studies. "The significance and incidence of folk medicine are as yet poorly understood and the underlying cultural factors inadequately studied." More recently, Welch, Comer and Steinman (1973:205) have said that links between the higher infant mortality rate, shorter life span, and higher incidence of tuberculosis of Mexican-Americans and traditional folk disease beliefs have been inadequately studied.

Methods

The three questions are studied through a survey of the literature on Mexican-American health beliefs and practices, use of professional health services, social structure, immigration patterns, and sources of folk disease beliefs. The literature comes from anthropology and the other social sciences, public health, and medical resources. The literature includes two basic types of studies: quantitative ones in which hypotheses are tested and descriptive studies with ethnographic material.

An Overview of the Literature

An "early" study of Mexican-American folk disease beliefs and practices was Lyle Saunders' sociological work, Cultural Differences and Medical Care which appeared in 1954 but was based on research done in the late 1940's. In the years that followed, several different approaches were undertaken to study Mexican-American folk diseases. Anthropological studies were done by Clark (1959), Rubel (1960, 1962, 1964, 1966), and Madsen (1964, 1969).

Kiev (1968) approached curanderismo as folk psychiatry for culture-specific psychiatric disorders. Torrey (1972) studied curanderos as a type of psychotherapist found in

Mexican-American communities using both anthropological and psychiatric foci. The study by Karno and Edgerton (1969) examined the extent that curanderismo acted as psychotherapy.

Anthropologists have studied folk-healing practices in native communities in Mexico for the most part as only one segment within the whole scope of an ethnography or study. These include, for example: Lewis (1960), Foster (1967), Romanucci-Ross (1973), and Friedman (1975), Redfield (1941) in The Folk Culture of Yucatan devoted a whole chapter to folk medicine and magic. Small sections on healing practices in different Indian groups appear in The Handbook of Middle Indians (1969).

Works that concentrate solely on folk disease concepts and cures in Mexico include: Foster (1951, 1953), M. Nash (1961), Metzger and Williams (1963), Holland and Tharp (1964), O'Nell and Selby (1968), C. and W. Madsen (1969), Turner (1970), Fabrega and Silver (1973), and Uzzell (1974).

J. Nash (1967) related social change to an increase in the number of curanderos (curers) and possible abuses of power by the curanderos in a Mayan community. Ingham (1970) took a structural approach to Mexican folk medicine.

Sociological studies of Mexican-American health practices include Jaco (1959, 1960) who focused on mental health, migration, and subcultural influences. Farge (1975) tested hypotheses by Madsen (1964), Rubel (1966), and Saunders (1954) among others. Other sociological studies include: Nall and

6

Speilberg (1967), and Welch, Comer and Steinman (1973).

Another category of literature includes primary research with statistics about health care patterns within Mexican-American communities. These studies come from a wide variety of sources: public health studies, health planning associations, medical journals, and nursing studies. They include: Anderson (1961), Creson, McKinley and Evans (1969), Baca (1969), Weiss (1969), Moustafa and Weiss (1968), Martinez and Martin (1966), Edgerton, Karno and Fernandez (1970), and Karno and Edgerton (1969).

Topics to be Covered

In order to evaluate the three questions, a number of topics are covered in this study. The sequence begins in the second chapter with information about the population under study: origins and characteristics of the Mexican immigrants, status of folk medicine in Mexico, origins of folk disease beliefs, and a brief survey of similarities and differences between Mexican and Mexican-American folk disease concepts.

The goals of the third chapter are to explore two topics: the five diagnostic categories: <u>susto</u>, <u>mal de ojo</u>, <u>empacho</u>, <u>caida de mollera</u>, and <u>mal puesto</u>; and the activities and characteristics of the Mexican-American curer (the <u>curandero</u>).

The fourth chapter investigates the first question: do Mexican-American folk disease concepts support traditional core values of the social system? This chapter has sections dealing with Mexican-American family structure, social networks, and traditional values and attitudes. The strategic roles illness plays in the community will be surveyed.

In the fifth chapter, the second and third questions are investigated. Subjects include: the social and cultural characteristics of individuals who believe in scientific health care, folk disease concepts, or both. Utilization of professional health care services is examined. This chapter contains statistical rather than descriptive data.

The final chapter sums up the results and conclusions about the three questions. Suggestions for future study are then offered.

CHAPTER II

MEXICANS AND MEXICAN-AMERICANS
CHARACTERISTICS AND DISEASE BELIEFS

Origins and Characteristics of Mexican Immigrants

It is estimated that four million Mexican-Americans reside in the United States (Grebler 1966:vi). Eighty-seven per cent reside in the Southwest (1960) with forty-eight per cent of them the sons or daughters of native parents. Thirty-nine per cent are of mexican stock. Of the thirteen per cent who live outside of the Southwest, six per cent are of Mexican ancestry while the other seven per cent are natives of native parents.

Mexican-Americans are a highly differentiated group in terms of socio-economic status. They also vary greatly in terms of regional variation. Groups of Mexican-Americans range from large barrios in metropolises such as Los Angeles to semi-rural or isolated colonias in the Southwest. Mexican-Americans range from recent immigrants to residents whose ancestors arrived in America several hundred years ago.

Distinctive features of the Mexican immigration include: greater number of males than females, heavy representation of laborers except farmers and miners, and an underrepresentation of professional, technical and managerial occupations (Grebler 1966:47-48).

Grebler (1966:81) makes several conclusions about the bulk of the immigration from Mexico. One, within Mexico, there is a continuous movement from rural to urban areas. Two, these people find it difficult to gain a foothold in the urban economy. Some of these people then emigrate to the United States. Mesa Centrale is an important source of immigrants although many immigrants come from border areas.

Statistics on the origins of Mexican immigrants are incomplete (Grebler 1966:21). Visas for emigres are most often issued in Tijuana, Cuidad Trujillo (Chihuahua), and the Central Plateau which includes a number of states such as Michoacan, Zacatecos, Jalisco, Coahuilla, and Durango.

Socio-Economic Patterns of Mexican-American Populations

Mexican-American populations are characterized by a great range of regional and social variation. Generally, there is believed to be two to three social classes.

In the California community of Sal si Puedes, residents claim that alta sociedad (high society) can be distinguished from the middle or lower class because the uppers are better dressed, have polite manners, speak better Spanish and English, and value education for themselves and their children (Clark 1959:18-19). This pattern represents a less structured pattern than the one found in New Mexico. (Gonzalez 1967:54). In New Mexico, ranked and stratified social classes have been a part of the total social structure since the beginning

10

of the Spanish-Colonial period. In those early times, the
upper class was small and composed of those of European
backgrounds. The lowest class was made up of Indians and
mestizos. The upper class was distinguished from the lower
class by the following criteria: lighter skin, better education, larger income, and more power in the political structure.

The middle class did not emerge in New Mexico until
after annexation. Today, the middle class is believed to be
the most anglicized. Members of this group speak English
in their homes, value education, and live in Anglo neighbor-
hoods (Gonzalez 1967:55). Madsen (1964) calls them
agringados or inglesados. In Sal si Puedes, it is the Mexican-
American upper class who have these characteristics (Clark
1959:18).

Mexicans: Origins of Their Folk Disease Beliefs

Mexican healing concepts are derived from a number of
sources. These sources include: early Greeks, Mediterranean
or Arab practices, Spanish (Catholic) beliefs, and customs
of pre-Conquest indigenous groups in the New World like the
Aztecs and the Mayans.

When the Spanish conquered the New World, Spanish medical
beliefs were largely based on classical Greek and Roman
practices. These had been adapted by Arab physicians such
as Rhazes (850-925 A.D.), Avicenna (980-1037 A.D.), and the
Spanish-Arabic physician, Avenzoar of Sevilla (973-1161 A.D.).

11

They were followers of the Hippocratic belief in four humors: blood, phlegm, black bile (melancholy), and yellow bile (choler). Each of the four humors was associated with specific characteristics: blood with hot and wet, phlegm with cold and wet, black bile with cold and dry, and yellow bile with hot and dry. Organs of the body were also believed to be hot or cold, wet or dry. For example, the heart was thought to be hot and dry. They believed the human body needed to maintain a balance between hot and cold, wet and dry. If the balance was disturbed, illness would result.

According to Foster and Rowe (1951:2), hot and cold were originally attributes of the four elements of ancient science: earth, air, fire, and water. Ingham (1970:85) traced the roots of the hot/cold opposition to pre-industrial Mediterranean cultures where hot was associated with consumption and cold with giving.

Today, the hot/cold dichotomy plays an important part in concepts of Mexican and Mexican-American disease causation. Disturbances in the balance between hot and cold are thought to be corrected by the ingestion of particular foods or herbs. The wet/dry dichotomy is no longer prevalent. (Foster and Rowe 1951:1).

The influence of Spanish Catholic beliefs is found in several forms in Mexican folk-curing ceremonies. (Foster 1953:203). Prayers are used for treatment. The curer often claims to have his powers based on the will of God. Spanish rulers considered good curers to be those who used traditional Spanish methods and called upon Catholic saints for assistance. Bones and unbroken eggs were recommended by the Spanish priests for curing diseases like the evil eye.

The effects of Catholic priests were less pervasive in Mayan villages of rural Mexico where the concept of the nagual (nawal) has continued to exist into the present time. In Tzeltal communities in Chiapis, belief in the nawal, an animal that is a source of curing or disease-producing power to its owner is still encountered. (Nash 1967:128).

Concepts about witchcraft are derived both from Spain and the New World. In Spain, Paracelsus, an influential physician prescribed burning waxen images for patients with excessive rage. He maintained that witches produced illness by shooting foreign bodies into the skin of their victims.

Spanish witches in the Old World were generally females vulnerable to severe punishments if caught. Among the magical techniques of Spanish witches was the ability to give the evil eye. Witches were believed to be allied with Satan. New World natives who used traditional curing techniques were believed by the Spaniards to be witches.

Sahugan (del Pozo 1967:66-68) stated that the Aztecs had two types of curers: the sorcerer and the physician. The sorcerer or witch was usually a man who had a pact with the Devil and could transform himself into an animal. Mexican-American folk disease concepts have maintained this division, the curer and the witch are not believed to be the same person.

Chronic diseases were viewed by the Aztecs as divine punishments for deviating from approved behavior. Catholic Mexican-Americans today sometimes believe that an illness may be a punishment from God.

According to Redfield, the Mayans had shaman-priests who had curing powers and powers of divining the cause of illness. (Redfield 1941:306). Curanderos in Mexican-American communities do not have priestly or religious functions unlike the Mayan curers.

Distribution of Mexican Folk Diseases

Mal de ojo (evil eye) is found today both in Spain and in the New World. The most widespread curing and divination technique for evil eye in Spain is to drop olive oil into water. This is rarely used in Mexico. Mexican-Americans use the egg cure for diagnosing evil eye.

Diseases like caida de mollera which involve displacement of organs is known in Spain and the New World. In both places, treatment is based on massage, poultices, and suction.

Susto or espanto (fright with soul loss) is found in Spain and in the New World. Susto is often caused by a strong emotional experience in Hispanic America while it is not a serious disease in Spain.

Extent of Folk Medicine in Mexico

There are several alternate systems of health care in Mexico. One is based on Western or scientific medicine and is supported by the federal government. The other system of beliefs is derived from folk concepts in Spain and the New World. These were discussed in the preceding sections.

In the Laguna (lake district) in Northern Mexico, (Southern Coahuilla and Durange), folk medicine flourished side-by-side with modern health services in the small, agrarian communities. In Torreon, a "modern, enterprising city", folk medicine was widespread. Kelly (1965:21) commented that in 1965, the people of the Laguna area had not yet been able to afford scientific medical services. Only those individuals with a high income could afford private (scientific) medical care.

In ejidos (small agrarian communities) in the Laguna area, health care was provided through the Servicios Medicos Rurales if the ejido paid its quota. The families in the community were free to use government medical services. Trucks conveyed sick people to the ejido hospital or to a curer who treated sorcery. Ejido funds paid for the curer and her medicines.

In some areas in Mexico, the federal government influenced practices of curers. In Huayapan (Morelos) during the 1940's, government nurses taught village curanderas how to use hypodermic needles and what patent medicines to prescribe.

15

The government installed a well-stocked infirmary in the home of one of Huayapan's curers. Curanderas in Huayapan currently used a combination of modern and folk techniques to treat clients (Friedlander 1975:98).

The Mexican government is extending scientific medicine into rural areas in two ways: every graduate of a medical school has to serve six months in a rural area and the Ministry of Public Health and Welfare has a system of free clinics which operate at the village level (Anderson 1961:268).

Inhabitants of rural areas in Mexico can use a curer who resides in the village and has the following attributes: complete control over causation and cure with approval of the supernatural, familiarity with the patient's social relationships, and ability to act as a mediator of problems in the social relations of the patient which are expressed through witchcraft-related diseases. (Fabrega and Silver 1973:199-203).

But villagers also seek out curers who reside in nearby towns or in cities. Sometimes, a famous charismatic curer is used. One such curer is El Nino Fidencio, a female curer who has a compound in Northern Mexico. Mexican-Americans also go to see El Nino Fidencio. Charismatic curers are not familiar with their patient's social relations and may do no more than touch the patient and say a prayer.

Relationships between disease causation, the curer, and the patient are changing in some areas in Mexico. In some areas, curers have lost their roles as agents of social control due to changes within the civil authority of the village. Witches or curers who practice witchcraft appear to be increasingly viewed as disruptive forces. In some areas, this has led to a high incidence of homicide involving curers or witches as victims (J. Nash 1967:458, Turner 1970:369).

The five diagnostic categories: _susto_, _caida de mollera_, _mal de ojo_, _empacho_, and _mal puesto_ are examined in Chapter III. Etiology, treatment, and curers are discussed.

CHAPTER III

MEXICAN-AMERICAN DISEASE BELIEFS AND CURERS

Four of the diseases discussed in this chapter are those selected by Rubel (1960) as an aggregate to resist anglicization. They are: susto, mal do ojo, empacho, caida de mollera, and empacho. A fifth disease, mal puesto is also included. Diseases are emically defined. A disease once labeled can be re-labeled at any time based on duration. Chronicity is associated with witchcraft-related illnesses. Shifting symptoms or resistance of the illness to treatment may result in the illness being re-labeled.

Madsen (1964:94) and Rubel (1966:170) contend that Mexican-Americans recognize two basic kinds of illness: natural and unnatural. A natural disease is one in which witchcraft is not involved in the etiology. Mal puesto is an unnatural (witchcraft-related) illness.

The etiologies of these folk illnesses involve both social relations and a condition of imbalance in the workings of the body. In this chapter, social relations as involved in the causation of illness are only briefly covered. In Chapter IV, the role of social relations involved in causation and curing of disease is considered at greater length.

Factors considered in the description of each diagnostic

category[1] are: precipitating occurrences, stages and symptoms. Methods of making the diagnosis and types of treatments are also considered. A discussion of folk curers occurs in the second section of this chapter.

Diagnostic Categories

Empacho

Empacho or "surfeit" is a stomach disorder which may occur because an individual eats too much of certain foods such as bananas, rice or potatoes. A hard "ball" develops inside the stomach. Sometimes empacho is believed to be caused by the failure to maintain a clean stomach. It's widely believed that good health is associated with periodic purgings of the intestinal tract and stomach (Saunders 1954:147).

Other causes of empacho relate to emotional experiences, constipation (an anglicized explanation), eating hot bread, overeating, an unpleasant experience, eating against one's will, or disliking what is eaten.

Symptoms of empacho are distended stomach, stomach ache, diarrhea, and vomiting. Treatment includes drinking fluids, specialized massage, snapping the skin on the back between the rib and kidney area, a cold medicine, or a mercury laxative to restore the system to equilibrium. A hot/cold treatment is to administer some form of cold metal such as quicksilver, then to administer a hot laxative such as castor oil.

Caida de Mollera

Caida de mollera or fallen fontanel refers to a disease which occurs in infants due to the "dropping" of the part of the head directly underneath the anterior fontanel. Causation may be related to bouncing the infant too vigorously, removing the nipple from the mouth too roughly so that the displaced or depressed fontanel causes the palate to protrude and inhibit eating.

Symptoms are vomiting, diarrhea, inability to eat, excessive crying, insomnia, lack of appetite, and dehydration in later stages.

One treatment involves attempting to push the protrusion back into place by pressing on the palate. Another treatment is to hold the infant by the ankles over a pan of water so that the tips of the infant's hair just touch the water. An adult may place his mouth over the baby's and suck. Herbs and raw eggs may be used to draw the fontanel back into place.

As a preventive measure, some babies wear tight caps to keep the fontanel or soft, boneless areas in the skull, in place.

Mal de Ojo

Mal de ojo or "evil eye" is caused by adults who have a strong glance. It usually occurs in children. Causation involves magic. The person who causes mal de ojo does so involuntarily (Baca 1969:217).

20

The strong/weak dichotomy is involved in mal de ojo.
The adult through strong glances inflicts illness because the
recipient, the child is weak.

An incorrect diagnosis or failure to cure mal de ojo
can lead to a terminal stage in the illness. The last stage
is a coughing fit so violent that the patient coughs up green
bile for which there is no cure.

Symptoms of mal de ojo are severe headaches, prolonged
weeping, fretfulness, high fevers, rashes, insomnia, and
nervousness.

Cures for mal de ojo vary according to the stage in the
illness. In an early stage, the individual who gave the
strong glance is asked to pass a hand over the forehead of
the victim. If the perpetrator can not be found than magic
and religious prayers are used. The patient may be rubbed
with hen's eggs to drain the power of the stronger person out
of the victim's body. The egg is then broken by the curandera
and put into a glass of water. The formation of the egg
indicates if the diagnosis of evil eye was correct.

Children wear bracelets or necklaces of pink coral as
protection against mal de ojo (Baca 1969:2173). Another
preventive measure is for the admirer to touch the head of
the child being complimented or admired.

Susto

One of the most prevalent folk diseases is susto or

fright which dislodges the soul from the body. Gillin (1948: 387) terms it "magical fright". Susto may occur when an individual is unable to cope with circumstances. According to Rubel (1966:162), susto occurs when someone is expected to perform adequately by the group but is unable to behave in the appropriate manner. A mother may get susto when her child gets mal de ojo or empacho, if she believes her child's illness could have been avoided (Kiev 1968:104).

Bracero informants listed the cause of susto as: seeing something which someone did not expect, a sudden surprise, unexpected news which caused a bad impression, to be scared by an animal, terror, and danger. Symptoms were said to be: nervousness, sleepiness, panic, weakness, and withdrawal from activities. The braceros listed such preventive measures as not getting excited, alertness, drinking water, and watchfulness (Anderson 1961:266-267).

Diagnosis is made by cleansing the body with an unbroken egg, then putting the raw egg into a glass of water to divine the cause of the illness from the egg's configuration.

The disease is cured by begging the soul to return, sweeping the victim with branches of a sweet-pepper tree, reciting Apostle's Credos, and calling the victim's name. Confession or discussion of the patient's life also occurs.

Mal Puesto

Both causation and curing of witchcraft-related diseases

involve what was termed as "sympathetic magic" by Frazer (Richards 1972:261). The underlying assumption is that things act on each other even at a distance because of a secret sympathy between them. Imitative magic is a form of sympathetic magic in which like influences like. In contagious magic, things which were once in contact with each other can continue to influence each other.

Saunders (1954:309) has suggested that in Mexican-American villages, belief in witchcraft has persisted relatively unchanged over the years. Witches have the ability to fly, change their physical form, influence the emotions of others, cause sickness, and even death. They work by casting spells, preparing and administering potions, polluting the air, poisoning food, using imitative magic (a doll) to harm another person.

Rubel (1966:168) contends mal puesto occurs because of three kinds of social relations: a spat between lovers, unrequited love, and invidiousness between individuals or families. Invidiousness is usually attributed to generalized others such as "the neighbors" or "someone".

According to Rubel, (1966:167), mal puesto has one symptom which is its exclusively: dramatic mania accompanied by the victim's belief that he is under someone else's control. Dramatic mania may be expressed as inappropriate laughing, self-mutilation, facial contortion, insomnia, and/or appetite disruptions. But Martinez and Martin (1966:63) found there was no one symptom which their informants could agree on for mal puesto.

Other symptoms of mal puesto are found in other diseases. These include: distended abdomen, loss of weight, coughing, pain, and conversations with invisible people.

If a disease becomes chronic, the family may examine the social relations of the victim to find the precipitating factor. Treatment involves having the victim accept the cause of his illness, destroying the doll, ingesting herbs or tonics, and using charms.

Curers

There are three main classes or types of curers within Mexican-American communities according to Rubel (1966:180). They include: housewives, neighborhood healers, and curanderos. Information in this section zeros in on the curandero since most of the information in the literature is on this class of curer.

It is not always possible to distinguish the curandero from the neighborhood curer. An individual may be identified as a curandero by some members of the community but not by others. For purposes of this paper, the curandero is defined as a Mexican or Mexican-American folk curer sought out by an aggregate larger than the family or neighborhood. The activities of the curandero include: defining the illness according to diagnostic categories which are accepted by the group and

prescribing or initiating treatment. The curandero receives
a gratuity or payment in exchange for his services. Treatment techniques include: injections, herbal remedies, prayers
to the saints, purgatives, massage, cupping, regulation of
the patient's diet, and advice on a particular course of
action.

Curanderos may come to their avocation in a number of
ways. The most frequent manner is through "the blessing of
God". Of his work, one curandero said, "God sent us these
afflictions and he also taught us how to cure them" (Madsen
1964:81).

Realization of curing power may begin with a mystical
experience...a sense oneness with something beyond the individual. One curandera described such an experience which
occurred when she was six or seven years old. Her dog died
and she felt a oneness with its body. She asked God to let
the dog live and it recovered. As a child she was a curer
and later in life became a curandera through an apprentice-
ship with an aunt who was a curer (Madsen 1964:90).

Voices, dreams, visions, or a feeling of understanding
towards sick people may inspire individuals to become
curanderos. Rubel (1966:186) suggests another factor which
validates the legitimacy of the curandero is a set of unusual
personality characteristics such as seizures, fainting, sleep-
walking, talk or singing while sleeping, or trances.

Clark (1959:163) characterizes a curandera as someone

who has more than the usual amount of lay knowledge of Mexican-American folk diseases. It is Clark's contention that curanderos do not have supernatural powers.

Curanderos vary considerably in educational background. The four curanderos Kiev (1968:30) studied in San Antonio ranged from the well-educated son of a physician to illiterate individuals who claimed no special powers. They were all born in Mexico and were highly religious.

According to Kiev (1968:31), the principal characteristic of curanderos is their religiousity. The powers of the curandero are derived from God, therefore if the curandero fails, it is theoretically not his failure but the will of God. In this way, the curandero is not held responsible.

Curanderos are often members of the same community in which their patients reside. They speak a common language. The vocabulary of the curandero includes few terms which are unfamiliar to the patient. The curandero sees patients in his own home except in emergencies. The healing process may begin with a social prelude, perhaps coffee and conversation. The curandero and the patient may discuss events in the barrio or village before the patient is examined. (Clark 1959:208).

In metropolitan areas, the behaviors of the curandero and patient may be different from that described in the preceding paragraph. In the study by Edgerton, Karno, and Fernandez (1970:128-129), the two curanderas studied, immediately launched into an examination of the patient. There was no social prelude.

Curanderos in Urban and Rural Areas

Recent studies have shown that curanderos reflect changes within Mexican-American communities. The curanderos described in the following paragraphs reflect differences in not only regional and individual variation but also rural or urban differences.

Rural Areas

Near Mexequito, Texas, Don Ramon, a charismatic curandero,[1] claims to have acquired his healing powers from the famous curer, Don Pedro Jaramillo because as a youth he dreamed about Jaramillo. Don Ramon believes his powers come from God through Jaramillo (Rubel 1966:190).

Don Ramon was born in Texas and went to Catholic schools. He lives in an expensive, multi-roomed house with a chapel which holds over two hundred people. Don Ramon conducts services which consist of Christian hymns and prayers, references to Jaramillo, and divination performed through ventriloquism by Don Ramon. Curing ceremonies are public. He touches diseased areas of the sick person and says prayers.

In Sal si Puedes[2] (near San Jose, California), Paula, a curandera has patients who reside within the same community she lives in. She charges little or nothing for her services and many regard her as a friend as well as a <u>curandera</u>. She sees patients in her home. Before diagnosis and treatment begin, there is a social interval of coffee and conversation. Paula bases her diagnosis on her knowledge of people in the community. She makes a diagnosis by taking the patient's pulse looking at his eyes or color, and palpating the troubled areas. She treats the ailment topically with herbs from her garden or gives the patient's relatives instructions on how to treat the patient. She welcomes suggestions from relatives of the patient on curing the patient (Clark 1959:207-208).

Saunders (1954:311) describes the activities of a <u>cur-andera</u> who treats a patient with a troubled marriage. The patient develops eczema because her husband is interested in another woman. The curandera diagnoses witchcraft done by the other woman and gives the husband a charm to protect him from the other woman. She gives the wife herbs to ensure her husband's affections, advice about making herself more attractive to her husband, a packaged skin preparation, and a vitamin B tonic. The treatment is successful, the husband returns to his wife and her skin clears up.

Urban Areas

"Mr. R." is a <u>curandero</u> in San Jose, California. He is seventy-five years old and has been a <u>curandero</u> for sixty-five years. He was born in Mexico. Among Mr. R.'s abilities are: power to treat physical and emotional illness, social and domestic problems, divine the future, pick winning numbers in Reno, Nevada; and get prisoners out of jail. He does his curing in his home which is filled with religious objects and presents from former patients. He accepts gratuities rather than setting fees. (Torrey 1973:143-144).

Torrey studied three of Mr. R.'s patients. All three went to see Mr. R. for help with marital problems. Two of them wanted divorces and were advised by Mr. R. to get divorces. Diagnosis of a folk disease was not involved (Torrey 1973:143-144).

Edgerton, Karno and Fernandez (1970:128) studies two curanderas in East Los Angeles. Both curanderas reflected the effects of acculturation of anglicization. One of the curanderas, Lupita charged five dollars for each treatment plus eight dollars for the remedy (cheap brandy). Lupita diagnosed a patient's illness as related to a stomach disorder and treated it with the brandy tonic, massage, and prayers.

The second curandera, Pilar, spoke Spanish with an American accent and frequently lapsed into English. She wore Western clothing and had her hair in curlers. She diagnosed a patient's symptoms as nerves then elicited facts about the patient's background, and counseled her on how to deal with her problems. Pilar recommended that the patient look for work, say a prayer daily, and light a votive candle to San Antonio. She charged two dollars for her services. (Edgerton, Karno and Fernandez 1970:128).

In the next chapter, concepts of disease and activities of curers are examined in the social contexts in which they occur. Traditional values and customs of Mexican-Americans are also discussed especially in respect to how they effect or are effected by ill health.

CHAPTER IV

DISEASE, HEALTH AND TRADITIONAL VALUES

This chapter investigates the first question posed:
do Mexican-American folk disease concepts support traditional
core values of the social system? The Mexican-American
family structure, and attitudes towards good health and
illness are examined.

Mexican-American Core Values in the Literature

Traditionally, the family of socialization is the most
important social unit in the barrio (Gonzalez 1967, Rubel
1966, Madsen 1964, Clark 1959, Saunders 1954). Rubel (1966:
55) classifies the nuclear family as the basic kinship unit
but there are many exceptions to this pattern. Most Mexican-
Americans would consider other relatives besides parents and
siblings as part of their familia. (Gonzalez 1967:43). An
individual's social unit may include his parents, his parents'
brothers and sisters, and his own brothers and sisters.

Respect for one's elders is a major organizing prin-
ciple of the Mexican-American family. Consanguinal and
affinal kin are bolstered by a ritual "kin" relation known
as the compradrazgo which is found among Catholic Mexican-
Americans. Special ceremonial bonds exist between a child's

parents and godparents. The compadres (co-parents) may be as close as brothers and sisters to the real parents. Compadres are consulted when trouble strikes, when advice is needed, and for assistance.

An individual's social relations center on real kin or fictive kin. Neighbors, instead of providing social outlets are, according to Rubel (1966:44) perceived as hostile. The family views itself as an island of security.

Gonzalez (1967:44) contends that studies done in urban and rural areas of New Mexico show that most actual social communication takes place between relatives. This supports Rubel's findings. Recent studies by Weaver (Gonzalez 1967:44) and Vincent (Gonzalez 1967:44) indicate that the extended family is still a viable unit.

The family has not escaped acculturation. The divorce rate has increased and the rate of intermarriage with Anglos has also increased. Children and parents frequently live in different areas. The Mexican-American family as a corporate, property-holding group has become disorganized because of the dispersal of family members in many areas (Gonzalez 1967:47).

The Mexican-American family is a bilateral kin group with what Gonzalex terms, a "patrilateral skew". Family relations are based on male dominance (Gonzalez 1967:47).

While the social relations of women are centered in the home, males are encouraged to associate with other males outside of the home. Young males belong to palomillas which

Rubel (1966:101) defines as a "network of informal dyadic relations between age-mates." There is no equivalent structure for young females.

Machismo is an idealized conception of masculinity which is based on a "florification of virility, strength, courage, and audacity (Torrey 1973:148).

Many individual's activities are overshadowed by the notion that the individual is not responsible for the outcome of his actions. Others outside the family have the ability to influence his life or punishments can come from God (castigo de Dios) (Kiev 1968:114, Torrey 1973:148).

Traditional Attitudes About Health

"Health is generally conceived of as a Gift of God, when a person becomes ill he is usually regarded as a passive, innocent victim of malevolent forces in his environment". (Fuentes 1972:124). A sense of personal responsibility for the occurrence of good or bad health is not held, according to Saunders (1954:152).

The view that Mexican-Americans see health as beyond their control was tested by Farge (1975:86). The sample was asked to respond to the statement, "Good health depends on good luck." Informants were drawn from three urban areas in Houston. One, the South County had a population of only 12.8 percent Mexican-Americans. The average educational level for the area was 12.5 years and the average income was $11,600.

The other two areas show great contrast. The Second Ward had sixty percent Chicanos with a median family income of $6,000 and a median education level of 7.9 years for formal education. The third area, Denver Harbor was fifty-five percent Chicano with a median family income of $7,240 and a similar educational level to the Second Ward.

In the second Ward, 39.2 percent of the residents agreed with the statement, "Good health depends upon luck" while 63.3 percent of the Denver Harbor area agreed with the statement. In the area with only a small Chicano population (South County), only 18.7 percent agreed with the statement. (Farge 1975:86).

Farge's study thus indicates that communities with larger Mexican-American numbers are more likely to maintain traditional attitudes toward health. But the study does not explain what causes the differences in percentage between the Second Ward and the Denver Harbor areas.

Mexican-American villagers in New Mexico and Colorado evaluated an individual's state of health not on external cues such as symptoms but on the ability of the individual to carry out his usual duties. If a man was not emaciated or in pain, he was not considered to be ill. Good health or strength was positively related to machismo (Schulman and Smith 1963:229-232).

Schulman and Smith (1963:229-232) found that Mexican-American villagers had three criteria for good health: absence of pain, a well-fleshed body, and a high level of physical activity. Healthiness was associated with strength and sickness with weakness (moral). Healthiness was also indicated by a sunny frame of mind, alertness and friendliness.

Traditionally, men are conceived of as stronger than women. The illness pattern bears this out. Children who are thought of as weak are susceptible to mal de ojo and caida de mollera. More women than men report incidents of susto (Rubel 1964, Uzzell 1974). Women are also frequently associated with witchcraft, both as the agent and the victim.

Mexican-Americans view illness as either caused by a lack of balance in the parts of the body such as a hot/cold imbalance or as caused by an upset in relations between the individual and his social or religious sphere (Madsen 1969:233). The aim of a course of treatment is not only to alleviate the sick person's symptoms but to correct the imbalance either in the body or in the social or religious sphere.

Role of the Family in Illness

Any study of Mexican-American folk diseases must emphasize the importance of the family in both diagnosing the illness, obtaining treatment for the illness, and curing the illness. Indeed, the family continues to be important in relations between the Mexican-American patient and Anglo health hear facilities. The Mexican-American patient seldom, if ever goes alone to a hospital or to see a physician (Clark 1959:231).

The illness sequence can be broken down into a number of stages which underscore the importance of the family (see Table 1). The order of the illness sequence is as follows: precipitating occurrence (causation) --- symptoms --- naming the diagnostic category --- selection of curer --- curer's diagnosis --- treatment. This is the order likely to be recounted by the patient. In reality, the precipitating occurrence may have occurred any time prior to the onset of symptoms and is frequently recalled only after the symptoms have appeared. The naming of the precipitating occurrence (fight with a neighbor, disagreement with mother-in-law, refusal to do something) may not come about until the patient has seen the curer.

Precipitating occurrences show wide variation. For example, a young child becomes ill. The parents wonder why the child has become ill and recall that a stranger complimented the child (precipitating occurrence). A curandero may be called upon or the parents may institute treatment for mal de ojo themselves.

A woman refused to loan her neighbor some corn. The woman became ill. She and her husband decide that her illness has been caused by witchcraft by the slighted neighbor (Rubel 1966:93-94).

Some folk diseases like mal puesto and susto may result from either interfamilial or intrafamilial troubles. Rubel (1966:171) suggests the Mexican-American family exists as an island of security in the midst of the invidiousness and threats of the outside world.

Rubel (1966:171) contends _mal_ _puesto_ does not involve members of a nuclear family but results from the activities of others outside of the family. In the literature, there are a number of instances of accusations of witchcraft by a daughter-in-law against a mother-in-law when they share the same household (Kiev 1968:111).

Madsen (1964:47) suggested that "the presence of an in-law living with members of a nuclear family almost always leads to a conflict in roles and a division of loyalties." Usually, the trouble lies with the mother-in-law/daughter-in-law dyad. The mother-in-law may either usurp her daughter-in-law's role or make demands on her son which supercede the wife's demands. One son said when giving in to his mother's demand to see a particular film, "What could I do? My mother who raised me had to see it. It made my wife mad and I'm sorry but she had no claim on me" (Madsen 1964:47). Several instances of witchcraft associated with mother-in-law/daughter-in-law relationships are found in the literature.[1]

Conflict between youth and age within the family is sometimes expressed in witchcraft accusations. In case two in Appendix A, conflict between the authority of the father and the disobedience of a grown son is ameliorated by accusations of witchcraft against a nonrelative, "a loose woman". The son is held unaccountable for violating the norm of obedience to the head of the family by casting the blame on the woman.

Demands made on a family member by other family members may be expressed in a folk disease when the member can not carry out the demands. A husband who is not <u>macho</u> but instead is dominated by his wife, develops <u>susto</u>.[2] A young boy does not follow his parents directions and his parents subsequently diagnose his fitful sleep as due to <u>susto</u>.[3]

TABLE I

Participants in the Illness

Naming the Precipitating Occurrence	Naming the Symptoms	Selecting the curer	Diagnosis	Treatment
sick person and/or family	sick person and/or family	sick person and/or family	curer, family	curer, family

Folk Diseases in Social Contexts

The occurrence of a folk illness may function to provide an excuse for behavior that is disapproved by the family and the community. Clark (1959:198-99) gives as an example of this, the case of a young man who breaks his engagement and then becomes ill. The man's behavior becomes understandable to others, the girl was a witch all along.

In another case, <u>susto</u> occurred in a woman who found family obligations to a brother and his family damaging to her own family's existence. Torn between the desire to help her brother and to meet her own family's needs, she became ill. Her neighbors, relatives, and a _curandera_ all diagnosed her illness as _susto_. Because she was ill, she was relieved of her obligations to her brother (Clark 1959:200-201)

A folk curer may mediate the squabbles of a husband and wife, not unlike an Anglo marriage counselor.

Giving a label such as _mal puesto_ or _susto_ to what the family or community perceives to be irrational behavior, provides both an explanation and a course of treatment for the affected individual.

Summary

In examining the relationships between traditional values, health attitudes, social relations, and folk illnesses, a number of patterns emerge. These diseases crosscut different segments of the Mexican-American population. In a great many instances, the precipitating occurrence of a disease involves either a family member or an "other". A large number of folk illness have etiologies related to troubles between family members or between neighbors. The occurrence of the folk disease often precipitates a solution to the trouble.

The occurrence of a folk disease often appears to coincide with a violation of a traditional value such as _machismo_ and obedience to the head of the house.

It is interesting to note that it is always adults who label the disease, not children. The illnesses discussed have symptoms that overlap so parents/adults often select a label on the basis of criteria other than symptoms.

In the following chapter, relations between disease beliefs and traditional values are linked to the effects of acculturation or "anglicization." Utilization of professional health care services by Mexican-Americans is also examined.

CHAPTER V

ACCULTURATION, HEALTH CARE, AND DISEASE BELIEFS

Introduction

The studies presented in this chapter come from a variety of sources but are mainly sociological or epidemiological. They sometimes present a bewildering array of data. In some cases, the studies confirm each other while in other cases, they contradict each other. In looking for similarities between the studies, the following facts emerge: the studies concentrate on narrow segments of the population both geographically and socioeconomically.

While the survey research from these studies provides a stunning amount of statistics, there is a lack of information about the social charactieristics of the communities in which the informants reside. Descriptive studies like those of Rubel, Madsen, and Clark present a wealth of detail about community life but lack statistics.

The one exception is the study by Farge (1975) which tested bypotheses by Rubel, Madsen, and Saunders on a large sample. But there is a problem here, too. While Rubel, Madsen, and Saunders studied rural areas, Farge concentrated on a metropolitan area.

The studies included in this chapter have the following

objectives: to explain underutilization of professional
health care services, to study the relationship between
retention of folk disease beliefs and the use of scientific
medicine, and the relationship between traditional Mexican-
American values and Anglo health care values.

Who Rejects Professional Health Care Services?

The study by Welch, Comer and Steinman (1973:210-212)
studied the variables involved in the retention of folk
disease concepts. These variables included: social characteristics (education, income, age, sex, and number of years
in the community) and attitude indicators related to closeness
to the Mexican-American society and culture (taking the inter-
view in Spanish, number of years of residence in the United
States, birthplace of parents, and the size of the Mexican-
American community).

Welch, Comer and Steinman (1973:210-212) found that
only one variable out of the nine was significant in deter-
mining resistance to using professional health care services:
size of the Mexican-American community. Those who resided in
a large Mexican-American community expressed resistance to
using Anglo health care facilities. But the authors found
that attitudes had little influence on actual health care
behavior. Health care behavior was more related to social
characteristics such as sex, age, income, and education.

In Nall and Speilberg's study (1967:304-304) of

tuberculosis patients in McAllen, Texas; three factors were found to be related to acceptance or rejection of the scientific treatment regime: marital status, presence of relatives in the neighborhood, and persons sought for advice on private matters. <u>Those married individuals who had spouses in the area and nearby relatives from whom they sought advice, more often rejected the treatment</u> (64 percent). Contradictorily, in Farge's study (1975:91), married and unmarried individuals did not have a significantly different health orientation, nor did medical orientation divide significantly according to family size.

Nall and Speilberg (1967:305) also found that <u>subjects who frequently visited with their neighbors were most likely to reject treatment</u>. This result is interesting in light of the contention by both Rubel (1966) and Madsen (1964) that female Mexican-Americans did not visit with their neighbors but restricted their social contacts to kin or fictive kin. Visiting with neighbors may represent an anglicized pattern, since visiting between neighbors is a frequent occurrence in Anglo communities.

In Nall and Speilberg's study (1967:305), age was directly related to the acceptance or rejection of scientific medicine. <u>Those informants over thirty-nine years old were more likely to reject treatment</u>. If retention of folk medical beliefs is associated with resistance to anglicization or acculturation, it would be expected that older informants would reject scientific medicine. Juveniles are exposed to public schools which stress not only Anglo values but scientific concepts about medicine, biology, physiology, and health.

The results of Farge's work (1975:86) conflict with the above data. He found that age was not an important predictor of health care attitudes but place of residence as a juvenile was. Place of residence in a rural area as a juvenile was associated with acceptance of folk beliefs and rejection of scientific medical beliefs.

Mexican-Americans who had traditional values[1] in Farge's study (1975:90), reported they would use a curandera if they needed help. This supports Rubel's promise that those who maintain traditional values, retain folk disease beliefs. But in Farge's study, scientific medical orientation failed to divide according to cultural congruence with the majority group. Consciousness of being a Chicano did not interact with medical orientation. Belief in folk diseases was not related to cosmopolitanism, sense of segregation, or scientific medical orientation.

Who Accepts Professional Health Care Services?

In the study by Creson, McKinley and Evans (1969:265), a moderate degree of acculturation was associated with acceptance of professional health care services.

In Farge's study (1975:169), the education variable

44

was an important factor in the acceptance of scientific medicine. <u>A higher education level was associated with a</u> <u>scientific medical orientation. Having a skilled job was</u> <u>associated with scientific health beliefs.</u>

Martinez and Martin (1966:162-164) studied seventy-five housewives in a low income housing project in a South-western urban area. Their median age was thirty-nine, they had an average of eight years of education, and two-thirds were born in the United States.

Thirty-three percent of the informants reported know-ledge of <u>mal puesto</u> while ninety-seven percent were familiar with the other four folk diseases used in the second question. Ninety-five percent reported the occurrence of one or more of the folk diseases in themselves, a relative, or an acquain-tance. There appeared to be no relationship between folk disease beliefs and such social characteristics as age, edu-cation, and place of birth except for <u>mal puesto</u>. Of eight reported cases of <u>mal puesto</u>, six were reported by women under the median age. A majority of the women were aware there were <u>senoras</u> (neighborhood curers) and a <u>curandera</u> in the neighborhood. More than half of the women in the sample had gone to <u>senoras</u> while only one-fifth had sought out a <u>curandera</u>. Eighty percent of the sample used physicians.

The study by Creson, McKinley and Evans (1969:264-266) like that of Martinez and Martin (1966), indicated <u>the same</u> <u>informants who had a good knowledge of folk diseases or went</u>

to curers also utilized professional health care services. The informants in the study by Creson, et. al., were interviewed in two hospital clinics: pediatrics and psychiatry. The subjects had low incomes, most were unskilled, one had a college degree. Only four of the subjects were born in Mexico. In two of the homes, English was spoken exclusively, while in the rest, Spanish took precedence. Forty-eight percent of the subjects had used a folk curer or a relative had. Eighty percent of the informants had a good knowledge of folk medicine including susto, mal de ojo, mal puesto, empacho, and caida de mollera. Some of the subjects regarded the neighborhood curers as "phonies" but said that curers elsewhere were honest.

Among bracero informants, physicians were utilized extensively while the herb doctor in camp was rarely used. Yet, many of the informants were able to define the folk diseases and recall instances of their occurrences. The informants were all males, low income, unskilled, and had little education. The bracero camp did not constitute a community. (Anderson 1961:122).

A physician in the Mexican-American community of Sal si Puedes stated that seventy-five percent of his patients asked questions about folk diseases although they had sought out scientific treatment (Clark 1959:209).

In Farge's study (1975:89-90), ninety-eight percent of the informants agreed with the following statement,

TABLE 2

Variables Related to Choice of Type
of Health Care by Mexican-Americans

1. Welch, Comer and Steinman (1973) - social character-
    istics (age, income, sex, education, number of years
    of residence in the community).

2. Nall and Speilberg (1967) - marital status, functioning
    family unit, relatives in the community, age.

3. Farge (1975) - socio-economic status, age, education,
    maintenance of Mexican culture, place of residence as
    a juvenile, self-determination, congruence with major-
    ity culture, preference for metropolitan area, sense
    of segregation.

4. Saunders (1954) - age, social characteristics.

5. Moustafa and Weiss (1968) - economic and social factors
    in urban areas, folk attitudes and beliefs in limited
    geographical areas.

6. Madsen (1964) - social class.

7. Rubel (1966) - Chicanismo, maintenance of traditional
    beliefs, resistance to anglicization.

8. Hoppe and Heller (1975) - familism, social class, and
    feelings of powerlessness.

"Medical doctors help people feel better." Belief in folk medicine was much less, the mean for the entire sample was 2.88 on a scale of zero to seven.

Moustafa and Weiss (1968:2) relate acceptance or rejection of professional health care services to social and economic factors in urban areas but in rural or "limited" areas, they contend folk medical beliefs and traditional values can influence acceptance or rejection of scientific medicine. They hypothesized that "As the Spanish-surname population represents a genetically heterogeneous group, we would expect that health and disease here are closely related to economic and social factors, as they are in other groups. In limited geographical areas, however, where a great measure of cultural homogeneity persists, attitudes and beliefs may influence behavior with respect to health practices and medical care to a point where differences in morbidity, disability, and perhaps even mortality become apparent." The evidence was not inconsistent with the hypothesis according to the authors.

Utilization of Professional
Health Care Services

In their study of an urban, Mexican-American sample in Nebraska, Welch, Comer and Steinman (1973:208) found that indicators of utilization of medical care were contradictory. Ninety-one percent of the sample stated they had a family doctor while fifty-one percent said there were times during the past year when they should have seen a doctor but had not. Seventy-two percent said they had never had a polio vaccination, sixty-one percent had never been vaccinated for tetanus.

Farge (1975:119) found that having preventive check-ups was positively related to a higher education level, higher income, and residence in a metropolitan area as a youth. These two studies indicate some support for Erasmus' hypothesis that preventive medicine is resisted in an effort to resist change while scientific medical treatments which produce observable changes are accepted (Erasmus 1952:426).

In Edgerton, Karno and Fernandez's work (1970:132) on an urban Mexican-American community in East Los Angeles, eighty percent said they saw a physician regularly and named the physician and his location. Mention of use of folk curers or folk illnesses did not rise as high as one percent.

Moustafa and Weiss (1968:46) hypothesized that negative attitudes towards Anglo institutions and a high level of belief in folk medicine was associated with a low use of professional health services. To support their hypothesis, they cited studies by Rubel, Madsen, and Saunders among others, and statistics on morbidity rates of Mexican-Americans as contrasted to other groups. This is similar to Rubel's two hypothesis as used in this paper.

The California Health Survey (1955-56) indicated a

lower rate of utilization of professional health care
services among Mexican-Americans. The Mexican-American group
had a rate of only 2.3 physician visits per year while Negroes
had 3.7 and Anglos, 5.6. Hospital admission rates reflect a
similar difference: seventy-six per thousand for Mexican-
Americans, eighty-two per thousand for Negroes, and ninety-
five per thousand for Anglos. "The aggregate days spent in
the hospital for non-maternity cases of Mexican-Americans
was only 608 per one thousand compared with 724 per thousand
for Negroes, and 827 per thousand for Anglos (Moustafa and
Weiss 1968:27-28).

In Colorado, for the year of 1960, the mean age at
death of persons living more than one year was 56.73 years
for Spanish-surnamed individuals and 67.46 years for others.
Neonatal death rate for Spanish-surnamed individuals in San
Antonio was 19.7. This was higher than Anglos (17.0) but lower
than non-Whites (23.7). (Moustafa and Weiss 1968:28).

Moustafa and Weiss (1968:28) contend that "Mexican-
Americans and Negroes have a closely comparable socioeconomic
status, so the differentials between these groups may be more
meaningful, whereas the differentials between Mexican-Americans
and Anglos in medical care utilization are probably more clearly
attributable to socioeconomic factors."

Weiss (1970) studied two Mexican-American communities
in California: Southeast San Diego and San Ysidro. The
bulk of the population in both areas claimed to use professional

health care services. The bulk of the population claimed to use professional health care services. Ninety percent of the respondents in Southeast San Diego and 86.5 percent of the respondent in the smaller Mexican-American community in San Ysidro said they used professional health care facilities.

TABLE 3

Percentage of Informants in the Same Sample
Who Have Folk Disease Beliefs and Use
Professional Health Care Services

	Nall and Speilberg	Martinez and Martin	Creson, et. al.	Farge	Welch, et. al.	Edgerton, et. al.
PHC	100[1] percent	80 percent	100[1] percent	71 percent	91 percent	80 percent
FDB	58 percent	95 percent	48-80 percent	2.88[2]	44 percent	<1 percent

	Weiss Southeast San Diego	San Ysidro
PHC	90 percent	86.5 percent
FDB	<7[3] percent	<7.2[3] percent

[1]Informants were interviewed while they were patients in a hospital or clinic.

[2]On a scale of 0 to 7.

[3]Category includes chiropractors and faith healers.

Utilization of Mental Health Care Facilities

Jaco (1959) and Madsen (1969) contend that Mexican-Americans are underrepresented in usage of mental health care facilities in Texas. Also in Texas (San Antonio), Kiev (1968) credited the success of curanderismo with curing psychological and emotional difficulties which in Anglo circles would have been treated by psychiatrists.

Edgerton, Karno and Fernandez (1970:125) found that Mexican-Americans were underrepresented in mental hospital populations. Ten percent of the population of California was Mexican-American in 1966, but only 3.3 percent were in mental hospitals. The authors stated that "education appears to be an important determinant of the nature of responses given to questions concerning mental illness" (Karno and Edgerton 1969:226).

A number of social and cultural variables have been utilized to account for the low number of Mexican-American mental patients. Jaco (1959:483) contended that underutilization of mental hospitals was the result of strength of the Mexican-American family which was associated with fewer mental dysfunctions.

Karno and Edgerton (1969:237) credited the following factors with a low incidence of Mexican-American psychiatric admissions to hospitals: language barrier, mental health role of the family practitioner, lack of facilities within Mexican-American communities, and the esteem-reducing nature of agency/client contacts.

According to Kiev (1968:179), curanderos are successful because they stress Mexican-American values: fatalism, adherence to traditional ways, acceptance of a mystical, non-rational view of the world, an emphasis on form and dignidad, and a reluctance to accept personal responsibility for troubles. These values clash with the values of Western psychotherapists.

The results of Wignall and Koppin (Moustafa and Weiss 1968:32) were contradictory. Wignall and Koppin studied admission rates to the state mental hospital in Colorado which provide over ninety-five percent of the total facilities for mental patients. The study found that general admission rate (1960-61) was significantly higher for the Mexican-American group. This was due to the high admission rate for males.

A study of first admissions to a New Mexico State Hospital (1958-59) also found that the first admissions rate for Mexican-Americans (41.8 percent) was higher than the Anglo rate (36.4 percent). While older persons had a higher rate of admission among Anglos, the opposite was true of Mexican-Americans (Moustafa and Weiss 1968:32).

It can be questioned at this point if mental hospital rates are influenced by cultural differences in the perception of mental illness. Behavior that is considered to be pathological by one culture, may be perceived as the norm in another culture. Meadow and Stoker (1965:276) examined the case files of 240 Mexican-American and Anglo hospitalized mental patients. "Behaviors reported by the Anglo hospital personnel in patient's case files were moderatley correlated with behaviors independently described by family members for both the Mexican-American and Anglo-American patient groups."

The results of Meadow and Stoker's work (1965:276) appear to indicate that there exists a common core of agreement between the members of the two cultures in the perception of deviant or pathological behavior.

Folk Disease As a Strategy to Resist Anglicization

The cases in Appendix B suggest the use of a folk disease to retain or renew the position of the individual within a traditional Mexican-American community. Cases five and six express outright resistance to acculturation. There is no data available to suggest that this is a widespread phenomenon.

Several cases indicate that professional health care services were used even though the subjects voiced considerable resistance to them. Sometimes, professional health care services were used after an individual has had his symptoms labeled as a folk disease and has accepted the diagnosis as accurate. The subjects in Appendix A, numbers eight and nine, became hospitalized psychiatric patients after they had believed their symptoms to be related to a folk disease.

Summary

The statistics on utilization of professional health

care services are highly contradictory. Researchers like Edgerton, Karno and Fernandez (1970); Weiss (1970), and Martinez and Martin (1966) report a high usage of professional health services by their informants (seventy to ninety percent). In contrast, statistics from state health surveys in three Southwestern states, reflect an underutilization of scientific medicine. Morbidity and mortality rates for these states also indicate an underutilization of scientific medical practitioners.

The picture for utilization of mental health facilities is also clouded. Statistics for California mental institutions reflect underutilization by Mexican-Americans while proportions for Mexican-Americans were higher in other Southwestern states than for other groups.

Acceptance or rejection of professional health care services was related to a complex number of variables in the literature. These variables included: familism, social class, feelings of powerlessness, size of the Mexican-American community, education level, type of occupation, presence of spouse, relatives, and neighbors; age, place of residence as a juvenile, level of acculturation, and income.

Belief in folk medicine or in traditional Mexican-American values was not a deterrent to either having a favorable attitude towards scientific medicine or to actually using professional health care services. The figures in Table 3 indicate that anywhere from less than one percent to ninety-five percent of the informants in seven studies believed in folk disease concepts or had a good knowledge of them while seventy-one percent or more of the _same_ informants had attitudes favorable to scientific medicine or used professional health care services.

CHAPTER VI

CONCLUSIONS

Summary

Mexican-Americans are a highly heterogeneous group in
both social and regional contexts. This is compounded by a
steady movement of Mexican-Americans from rural to urban
areas. Health care beliefs show changes in both the United
States and Mexico. Two belief systems are available in many
areas of Mexico: professional health care services and folk
curers. In some areas, individuals use both systems. Other
areas show the effects of the influence of scientific medical
concepts on folk curing techniques and on curers.

Causation, symptoms, and remedies for the five folk
diseases (susto, mal de ojo, empacho, caida de mollera, and
mal puesto were consistent with traditional Mexican-American
values such as machismo, and respect for elders.

Curers (curanderos or neighborhood curers) often
reflected values that were the same as those of their patients.
Some curers treated their patients on the basis of their own
knowledge of the community when they lived in rural areas.
In contrast, some curanderos in urban areas, had anglicized
characteristics. These curers often treated their patients
for troubles which had not been transformed into folk illness

such as <u>mal</u> <u>puesto</u> or <u>empacho</u>. Curers treated their patients for marital problems or, for example, "nerves".

Many occurrences of folk diseases in non-urban areas involved precipitating agents of the illness who were outside of the family such as schoolmates, neighbors, employers, and others. The traditional Mexican-American family played a prominent part in the occurrence of a folk disease. They frequently determined the nature of the disease and the pre-cipitating occurrence, in addition to selecting the curer and helping in the treatment. In some instances, the curer, whether a relative, a neighbor, or a curandera acted as a mediator between the sick person and others.

Acceptance or rejection of professional health care services was related to a complex number of variables in the literature. Variables associated with resistance to profes-sional health care services were: residence in a large Mexican-American community, lack of skilled occupations, low educational level, closeness to spouse, relatives (in resi-dence), older age, residence in a non-urban area as a juvenile.

Acceptance of professional health care services was associated with the following variables: moderate accultura-tion, higher education level, higher income, skilled occupa-tion, younger age, and preference for residence in an urban area.

Informants often had a good knowledge of folk diseases and treatments, saw curers and used professional health care services. Health care beliefs may be compartmentalized.

There is some indication that Mexican-Americans under-
utilize professional health care services but it has not
been determined if the cause is solely based on socioeconomic
factors.

Conclusions

Question 1 - Do Mexican-American folk disease concepts support
traditional core values of the social system?

The literature showed a clearcut relationship between
traditional values and folk diseases.

Question 2 - Do traditionally-oriented Mexican-Americans
retain beliefs in the five folk diseases and is this associated with resistance to Anglicization?

Belief in the five folk diseases (susto, mal de ojo,
mal puesto, empacho, and caida de mollera) varies considerably
from high to low in the survey research studies (from less
than 1 percent to 95 percent). In some studies, a high score
on Maintenance of Mexican Culture was associated with belief
in folk diseases. But the studies also indicated that resistance to use of professional health care services or belief
in scientific medicine were not related to Chicanismo or
belief in folk diseases. Tentatively, it can be said that
traditional Mexican-Americans who believe in folk diseases
do not use their beliefs to resist scientific medicine. The
literature suggests that scientific medicine and folk medicine

may be used concurrently or consecutively.

Question 3 - Is retention of folk disease beliefs associated with underutilization of professional health care services is contradictory. There is some suggestion that professional health care services are underutilized but the factors involved in this are numerous and sometimes contradictory. These factors involve cultural variables, socioeconomic variables, or possibly past experiences with professional health care services.[1]

It can not be said that Rubel's two hypotheses (page two) have been proved. Some of the literature suggests that although belief in traditional values and folk diseases are associated this does not necessarily lead to resistance to anglicization or rejection of Anglo health care services. Socio-economic factors or other factors are, in urban areas are involved in a possible underutilization of professional health care services has not been clearly defined by the literature.

Suggestions for Future Study

To evaluate the effect of cultural factors (such as traditional values) on utilization of professional health care services, a study should include the following characteristics:

1. examination of urban and rural areas

2. informants in the study are matched for

60

socioeconomic and cultural characteristics

    3.   examination of contexts within which Mexican-American folk diseases occur

    4. a study of the influence of urbanization or acculturation on folk disease concepts and curers

Questions to be answered by the proposed study include:

    1. Do traditional Mexican-Americans use professional health care services less than acculturated Mexican-Americans?

    2. Does underutilization occur in urban areas, in rural areas, or in communities with high cultural homogeneity?

    3. What are the social and cultural characteristics of Mexican-Americans who use professional health care services?

    4. What are the social and cultural characteristics of Mexican-Americans who do not use professional health care services?

A Final Note

In concluding this paper, it is worthwhile to recall that folk disease concepts reflect social conflicts rather than events in nature (Ackerknect 1971:169). Scientific medicine, in contrast, deals with bacteria, germs, and genes which are neither friendly nor hostile. Scientific medicine is not based on the Hippocratic notion of humors. Illness caused by an imbalance between heat and cold is not a viable concept in scientific medicine. Folk medicine deals with the personal, scientific medicine with the impersonal.

Scientific medicine may infringe on traditional Mexican-American customs and values without even being aware of it. Modern or Western medicine is just beginning to take cognizance of Mexican-American values, the importance of modesty, the strong role of the family in illness occurrences, folk disease beliefs, and causal factors in illness which are not scientific but correspond to conflicts or values within the Mexican-American community.

APPENDIX A

Cases of Folk Illnesses in the Literature

1. A male Chicano was justifiably fired for failure to show up for work. He told his palomilla that he had been wronged and was going to demand to be reinstated. On the way to see his former employer, he tripped and fell. The next day, he developed susto. He was treated by a neighbor who did curing. She ordered him to bed for several days thus avoiding the consequences of his boasts. (Madsen 1964:98).

2. A son first went out with a "loose woman" instead of delivering furniture for his father. Later, he went to deliver the furniture and smashed up the truck. His mother found a small ball of cloth inside the son's shirt with a chunk of clay in it. The mother deduced that the son's misbehavior was the result of being bewitched by the "loose woman". (Madsen 1964:99)

3. A husband and wife fought because the wife suspected her husband was seeing another woman. The husband threatened his wife with a knife and then accidentally cut himself on the hand. The husband developed growths on his head and the wife's hand developed sores. They went to physicians and then to a fortuneteller who informed them that someone else had caused their troubles because of envy. (Rubel 1966:88).

4. A woman had abdominal swelling for several years. Doctors could not cure her. The woman and her husband then decided that illness was caused by neighbors whom the woman had refused to give corn. The husband threatened to kill the neighbors and actually tied them up but his wife did not get better. The husband punctured his wife's abdomen and a yellow liquid the color of corn came out. She was cured. (Rubel 1966:93-94).

5. A man became infatuated with a neighbor's daughter. His machismo was threatened when it developed that she was not interested in him. The girl became ill and went to a hospital. Her parents went to a curandero who told them to dig up two dolls in a cemetery. They did what the curer told them to do and the girl was cured. (Rubel 1966:95)

6. A young couple got married. The girl's aunt did not like the groom. It was an unhappy marriage so the couple went to see a curer who told them they would have to overcome the malice of someone who had not wanted them to get married. The marriage was more successful after that. (Rubel 1966:96)

7. a husband beat up his wife several times so she went to live with her mother-in-law but they also fought. The wife began to see another man and the husband saw another woman. The wife had a "nervous breakdown" and believed she was bewitched. She was taken to a curandera but failed to get better. She was placed in a mental hospital. (Kiev 1968:115)

8. A husband believed that homosexuals were threatening to assault him. As a boy, he had been passively involved in a number of homosexual incidents. After he married, he lived in his mother's house with an aggressive wife who repeatedly criticized him for being shy. He developed susto. (Kiev 1968:119-120)

9. A wife blamed her illness on bewitchment caused by her mother-in-law. When the wife had gone to take care of her sick father, her husband went to live with his mother. The wife believed her mother-in-law had bewitched her so that she would return to her husband. (Kiev 1968:109-110)

10. An Arizona rancher shot a woman because, he claimed, she was a witch who had sprinkled powder on his wife and caused her to go blind. No curer was able to help his wife. (Saunders 1954:308)

11. A man in Mexiquito, Texas, believed his neighbor had caused the death of his wife through witchcraft. He attempted to take the case to court but his wife was dead and there was no admissable evidence. (Rubel 1962:164)

12. Ricardo, a five year old boy went on a picnic at a lake with his family. They urged him to go into the water but he refused and went to sleep instead. He slept fitfully during the night. The next morning, his family decided he had been asustado (the condition of being ill with susto) the previous day. Susto occurred because the family demanded that the boy enter the water and he was unable to accede to their demands. The family took the boy to a neighboring woman to be cured. (Rubel 1960:805)

13. Mrs. Benitez had a seizure after having an argument with her son-in-law. She had refused to give him his gun and he criticized her rudely and assaulted her daughter. The next day, Mrs. Benitez had a susto attack. (Rubel 1960:806)

14. Miguel boasted to his peers that he would conquer Margarita at a dance but he then discovered that his older brother had designs on the same girl. His peers were expecting to see him "conquer" the girl. Miguel brooded and the day before the dance, he noticed a pain in his leg. His mother diagnosed the pain as due to aire[1] and sent him to bed. He was not able to go to the dance. (Madsen 1964:97-98)

15. Juanita was caught shoplifting by an Anglo store manager. He threatened her with arrest and called her "a thieving Mexican" before he let her go. She did not tell her family about her experience. Later in time, Juanita refused to marry her suitor. Then, she began to act "strangely" and said a demon was following her in order to destroy her soul. When left alone, Juanita became hysterical. She cried frequently. Her family explained her behavior as due to witchcraft caused by a rejected suitor. (Madsen 1969:236).

16. A young woman expecting her first child became angry with her husband when he came home drunk. She scolded him so he beat her and put her out of the house in the rain. She walked in the rain to her parents' house and told them what had happened. They took her to a curandera because they were afraid her unborn child would later suffer from susto. News of the husband's behavior spread through the barrio and the husband was criticized, not for beating his wife but for endangering the life of his unborn child. He was persuaded to apologize to his wife. (Clark 1959:198-99)

17. An elderly woman was admitted to a hospital against her wishes. When her illness had improved, she was forced to take showers every day by the nurse despite her objections. She was used to taking baths at less frequent intervals. One day, coming back from the shower, she had an attack which she identified as mal aire (bad air). Her relatives brought her some herbs marinated in oil to massage the affected area. (Clark 1959:202)

APPENDIX B

Cases of Folk Illnesses in the Literature Related to Acculturation

1. A daughter who was well-educated became a bookkeeper and a notary. She stopped eating all together and subsequently died at the age of twenty-three. Her mother believed her death was due to mal puesto caused by someone's envy of her daughter. (Rubel 1966:96-97)

2. Roberto was from an inglesado (anglicized) family but his schoolmates were not. He did well in school unlike his peers but did not make friends. Suddenly, he began to flunk courses. He then made friends. He wanted to marry but both sets of parents refused to give permission. The girl refused to see him again. His friends laughed at him and his face broke out in acne. Roberto went to a curer to be treated for bewitchment. (Madsen 1964:99-100)

3. Jose became a television repairman. He then decided to buy an automobile and asked his parents to give him permission. They refused. He had already told his palomilla he was going to buy the car. Jose moved out of his parents' house and bought the car. He began to use Anglo mannerisms in both Anglo and Latin social contexts. The mother of a Latin girl believed Jose had made an improper suggestion to her daughter when he came to repair a television. His reputation was ruined and his services as a repairman were requested less and less. He could not pay for his car payments and it was repossessed. Jose began to believe an evil force had taken over his life. He went to a curandero who told him he was bewitched and to be cured he would have to renew his relations with his family. (Madsen 1964:100-102)

4. Maria's husband began an extramarital affair and spent his money outside of the family. Maria wanted to take a job to make up for the missing money. Her husband refused to give permission and Maria then refused to accompany him when he went North to pick crops. She took a job, began secretarial classes, adopted anglicized mannerisms, and ignored her family. When her husband returned, Maria was ill with what a curandera

66

diagnosed as witchcraft. The husband conferred daily with the curer. The curer pointed out the husband's misbehavior when the husband's mother was present, so the husband was not able to blame his wife for everything. The curer got the wife to beg her husband's forgiveness. The wife resumed her role within the family in a humble and subdued manner. (Madsen 1964: 102-104)

5.   A grandmother born and reared in Mexico, claimed that she had suffered from stomach trouble since moving to the United States. She related the cause of her illness to "artificial food" which she was forced to eat in America. She told her American-born children and grandchildren that she had been healthy in Mexico but the United States was making her ill. (Clark 1959:201)

6.   A middle-aged woman attributed her chronic poor health and ability to conceive only one child to both an abdominal operation and the semi-raw food she had eaten in the United States. After she moved from a rural area in Arizona to urban San Jose, she attributed her poor health to the rapid pace of her new life. (Clark 1959:201-202)

NOTES

Chapter III

1. Charismatic curers frequently do not establish a personal realtionship with the sick person. They may not delve into the social relationships of the patient.

2. Sal si Puedes translated means, "get out if you can".

Chapter IV

1. See Appendix A, numbers 7 and 9.

2. See Appendix A, number 8.

3. See Appendix A, number 12.

4. See Appendix A, number 15.

Chapter V

1. They scored strongly on the measure, Maintenance of Mexican Culture.

Chapter VI

1. This factor has not been tested in the literature.

Appendix A

1. _Aire_ is caused by a hot/cold imbalance in the body.

REFERENCES CITED

Ackerknecht, E.
    1971   Primitive Medicine's Social Function. In
            Medicine and Anthropology: Selected Essays.
            H.H. Walser and H.M. Koebling, eds., Pp. 167-
            171. Baltimore: The Johns Hopkins Press.

Adams, Richard N. and Arthur J. Rubel
    1967   Sickness and Social Relations. In Handbook of
            Middle American Indians, 6. Manning Nash, ed.
            Pp. 333-356.

Anderson, Henry
    1961   The Bracero Program in California. Berkeley:
            University of California Press.

Argondona, Mario and Ari Kiev
    1972   Mental Health in the Developing World. New
            York: The Free Press.

Baca, Josephine
    1969   Some Health Beliefs of the Spanish-Speaking.
            American Journal of Nursing, 69:2172-2176.

Carrasco, Pedro
    1969   Central Mexican Highland: Introduction. In
            Handbook of Middle American Indians, 7. Evon
            Z. Vogt, ed. Pp. 579-601. Austin: University
            of Texas Press.

Clark, Margaret
    1959   Health in the Mexican-American Culture. Berkeley:
            University of California Press.

Creson, D.L., Cameron McKinley, and Richard Evans
    1969   Folk Medicine in the Mexican-American Subculture,
            Diseases of the Nervous System 30:264-266.

Currier, Richard L.
    1966   The Hot-Cold Syndrome and Symbolic Balance in
            Mexican and Spanish Folk Medicine. Ethnology
            5:251-263.

DeCicco, Gabriel
    1969   The Chatino. In Handbook of Middle American
            Indians, 7. Evon Z. Vogt, ed. Pp. 360-366.
            Austin: University of Texas Press.

del Pozo, Efren C.
    1967   Empiricism and Magic in Aztec Pharmacology. In
            Ethnopharmacologic Search for Psychoactive Drugs.
            Bo Holmstedt and Nathan S. Kline, eds. Pp. 59-
            76. Public Health Service Publication. U.S.
            Printing Office.

Edgerton, Robert B., Marvin Karno and Irma Fernandez
    1970   Curanderismo in the Metropolis. American Journal
            of Psychotherapy 24:124-134.

Erasmus, Charles
    1952   Changing Folk Beliefs and the Relativity of
            Empirical Knowledge. Southwestern Journal of
            Anthropology 8:411-428.

Fabrega, Horacio, Duane Metzger, and Gerald Williams
    1970   Psychiatric Implications of Health and Illness
            in a Maya Indian Group. Social Science and
            Medicine 3:609-626.

Fabrega, Horacio and Daniel B. Silver
    1973   Illness and Shamanistic Curing in Zinacantan,
            An Ethnomedical Analysis. Stanford: Stanford
            University Press.

Farge, Emile J.
    1975   La Vida Chicana: Health Care Attitudes and
            Behavior of Houston Chicanos. San Francisco:
            R and E Research Associates.

Foster, George M. and John H. Rowe
    1951   Suggestions for Field Recording of Information
            on the Hippocratic Classiciation of Diseases
            and Remedies. Kroeber Anthropological Society
            Papers 5:1-3.

Foster, George M.
    1953   Relations between Spanish and Spanish-American
            Folk Medicine. Journal of American Folklore
            66:201-217.
    1967   Tzintzuntzan. Boston: Little, Brown and Co.

Frake, Charles
    1961   The Diagnosis of Disease Among the Subunum of
            Mindinao. American Anthropologist 63:113-132.

Friedlander, Judith
      1975   Being Indian in Hueyapan. New York: St.
              Martin's Press.

Fuentes, Jose
      1972   Please Doctor, Listen to Me. In Viva La
              Diferencia. Manual Ferran, ed. Albuquerque:
              Regional Medical Programs Services.

Gillin, John
      1948   Magical Fright. Psychiatry 11:387-400.

Gonzalez, Nancie
      1967   The Spanish Americans of New Mexico: A Distinc-
              tive Heritage. Mexican-American Study Project,
              9. Los Angeles: University of California Press.

Grebler, Leo
      1966   Mexican Immigration to the United States: The
              Record and Its Implications. Mexican-American
              Study Project, 2. Los Angeles: University of
              California.

Holland, William R. and Roland G. Tharp
      1964   Highland Maya Psychotherapy. American Anthro-
              pologist 66:41-52.

Hoppe, Sue Keir and Peter L. Heller
      1975   Alienation, Familism and the Utilization of
              Health Services by Mexican-Americans. Journal
              of Health and Social Behavior 16:304-314.

Humphrey, Norman D.
      1945   Some Dietary and Health Practices of Detroit
              Mexicans. Journal of American Folklore 58:
              255-258.

Ingham, John M.
      1970   On Mexican Folk Medicine. American Anthropol-
              ogist 72:76-87.

Jaco, E. Gartly
      1959   Mental Health of the Spanish-Americans in Texas.
              In Culture and Mental Health. Marvin K. Opler,
              ed. New York: the MacMillan Company.

Karno, Marvin and Robert B. Edgerton
      1969   Perception of Mental Illness in a Mexican-
              American Community. Archives of General Psy-
              chiatry 20:233-238.

Kelly, Isabel
    1965   Folk Practices in Northern Mexico. Austin:
            University of Texas Press.

Kiev, Ari
    1968   Curanderismo, Mexican-American Folk Psychiatry.
            New York: The Free Press.

Madsen, William
    1964   Mexican-Americans of South Texas. New York:
            Holt, Rinehart and Winston, Inc.
    1969   Mexican-Americans and Anglo-Americans: A
            Comparative Study of Mental Health in Texas.
            In Changing Perspectives in Mental Health.
            F. Plog and R. Edgerton, eds. New York: Holt,
            Rinehart, and Winston, Inc.

Madsen, William and Claudia Madsen
    1969   A Guide to Mexican Witchcraft. Mexico City:
            Editorial Minitiae.

Martinez, Cervando and Henry W. Martin
    1966   Folk Diseases Among Urban Mexican-Americans.
            Journal of American Medical Association 196:
            161-164.

Meadow, A. and D. Stoker
    1965   Symptomatic Behavior of Hospitalized Patients.
            Archives of General Psychiatry 12:267-277.

Moustafa, A. Taher and Gertrud Weiss
    1968   Health Status and Practices of Mexican-Americans.
            Mexican-American Study Project. Advance Report
            11. Los Angeles: University of California
            Press.

Nall, Frank C. and Joseph Speilberg
    1967   Social and Cultural Factors in the Responses of
            Mexican-Americans to Medical Treatment. Journal
            of Health and Social Behavior 8:299-308.

Nash, June
    1967   Death As a Way of Life: The Increasing Resort
            to Homicide in a Maya Indian Community 69:455-
            470.

Nash, Manning
    1967   Witchcraft As a Social Process in a Tzeltal
            Comminity. In Magic, Witchcraft and Curing.
            John Middleton, ed. Garden City: The
            National History Press.

O'Nell, Carl W. and Henry A. Selby
    1968   Sex Differences in the Incidence of Susto in
            Two Zapotec Pueblos: An Analysis of the
            Relations Between Sex Role Expectations and a
            Folk Illness. Ethnology 7:95-105.

Ravicz, Robert and A. Kimball Romney
    1969   The Amuzgo. In Handbook of Middle American
            Indians, 7. Evon Z. Vogt, ed. Pp. 417-433.
            Austin: University of Texas Press.

Redfield, Robert
    1941   Folk Cultures of Yucatan. Chicago: University
            of Chicago Press.

Romanucci-Ross, Lola
    1973   Conflict, Violence and Morality in a Mexican
            Village. New York: National Press Books.

Richards, Cara
    1972   Man in Perspective. New York: Random House.

Rubel, Arthur J.
    1960   Concepts of Disease in Mexican-American Culture.
            American Anthropologist 62:795-814.
    1962   Social Life of Urban Mexican-Americans.
            Doctoral Dissertation. University of North
            Carolina.
    1964   The Epidemiology of a Folk Illness: Susto in
            Hispanic America. Ethnology: 3:268-283.
    1966   Across the Tracks, Mexican-Americans in a
            Texas City. Austin: University of Texas Press.

Saunders, Lyle
    1954   Cultural Differences and Medical Care. New York:
            Russell Sage Foundation.

Schulman, Sam and Ann M. Smith
    1963   The Concept of Health Among Spanish-Speaking
            Villagers of New Mexico and Colorado. Journal
            Of Health and Human Behavior 4:226-234.

Torrey, E. Fuller
    1972   The Mind Game. New York: Bantam Books.

Turner, Paul
    1970   Witchcraft as Negative Charisma. Ethnology
            9:368-372.

Uzzell, Douglas
    1974   Susto Revisited: Illness at Strategic Role.
            American Ethnologist 1:369-378.

Weiss, Gertrud
    1970   Southeast San Diego Health Study. San Diego:
              Comprehensive Health Planning Association of
              San Diego Imperial Counties.

Welch, Susan, John Comer and Michael Steinman
    1973   Some societal and Attitudinal Correlations of
              Health Care Among Mexican-Americans. Journal
              of Health and Social Behavior. 14:205-213.

Young, Alan
    1976   Some Implications of Medical Beliefs and
              Practices for Social Anthropologists.
              American Anthropologist. 78:5-22.